GALVESTON DIET COOKBOOK

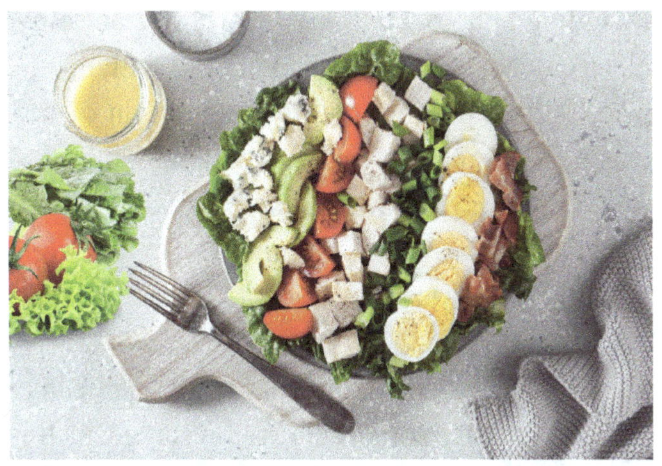

Unleash Your True Potential with Nourishing and Delectable Recipes to Ignite Fat Loss, Balance Hormones, and Boost Your Vitality

Dr. Jaclyn N. Anderson

TABLE OF CONTENTS

INTRODUCTION

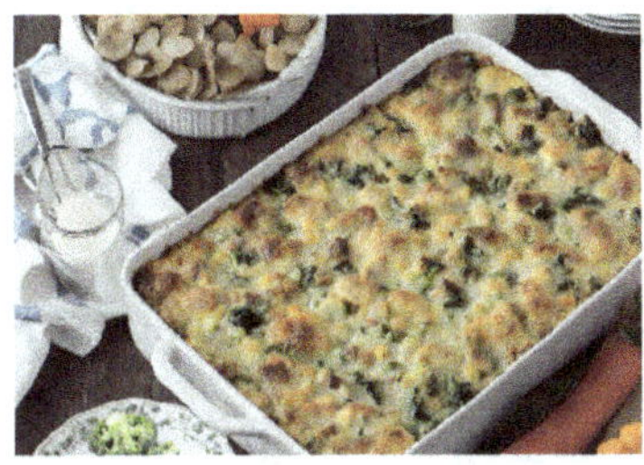

Women undergoing midlife encounter numerous physical changes, including hormonal shifts, metabolic variations, and lifestyle adjustments that often lead to weight gain, inflammation, and potential health issues. However, specific strategies can help bolster their health during this crucial phase. The Galveston diet is specifically tailored for women aged 40 and above, prioritizing a well-rounded diet, regular exercise, and self-care to stabilize hormones, reduce inflammation, and manage weight effectively.

Polycystic Ovary Syndrome (PCOS) is a prevalent endocrine disorder affecting about 1 in 10 women, especially those who are overweight or obese. It's characterized by irregular menstrual cycles, increased levels of male hormones (androgens), and the development of multiple ovarian cysts, which can hinder conception and lead to weight gain and various health concerns. Maintaining a healthy body weight is crucial for women managing PCOS, as excess weight can worsen symptoms and elevate the risk of complications like diabetes, hypertension, and heart diseases.

The Galveston diet program offers potential support to women dealing with PCOS by focusing on weight loss and holistic well-being. Through a balanced, nutrient-rich diet, regular exercise, and self-care practices, women with PCOS can improve their health, alleviate symptoms, and enhance their overall condition. By embracing this program and integrating healthy habits into their daily lives, women can feel more confident and empowered in managing their health while navigating the changes of midlife. The Galveston diet serves as a structured framework that provides guidance and support to achieve various health objectives, whether it's weight loss, reducing inflammation, or enhancing overall well-being.

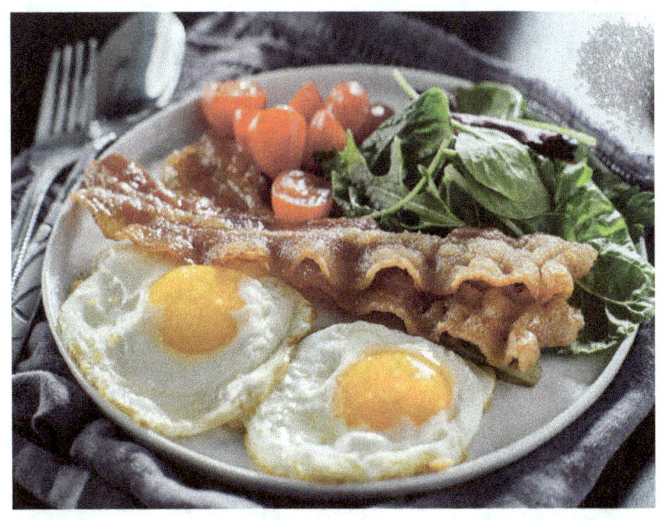

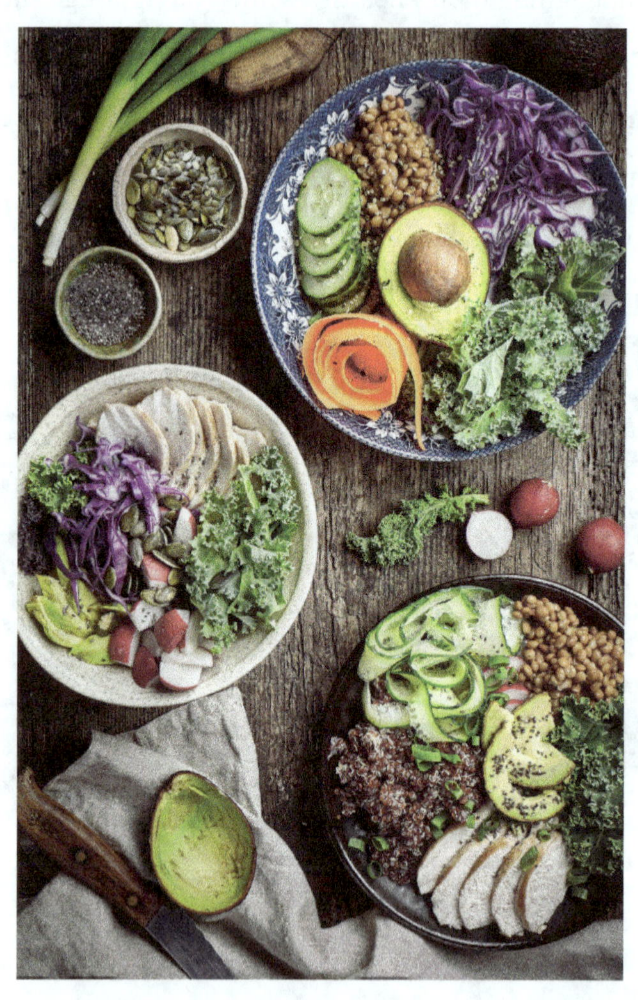

CHAPTER 1:

UNDERSTANDING THE GALVESTON DIET

What Is Galveston Diet

The Galveston Diet is a specialized nutritional approach tailored for women navigating menopause or perimenopause. Developed by Dr. Mary Claire Haver, an OB-GYN, it aims to address the unique challenges women face during this phase of life, specifically focusing on hormonal changes and their impact on weight and overall health.

Principles of Galveston Diet

1. **Hormonal Balance:** The diet aims to restore hormonal equilibrium, particularly targeting insulin and cortisol levels. It emphasizes foods that help

regulate these hormones, aiding in weight management and overall health.

2. **Low Inflammatory Foods:** The diet encourages the consumption of anti-inflammatory foods, such as leafy greens, fatty fish, and healthy fats, while minimizing inflammatory foods like refined sugars and processed items.

3. **Intermittent Fasting:** Incorporating intermittent fasting, particularly overnight fasting, is a central aspect of the Galveston Diet. This fasting window helps regulate insulin and supports the body's natural healing processes.

4. **Nutrient-dense Foods:** Emphasis is placed on nutrient-dense, whole foods that offer a range of vitamins, minerals, and antioxidants to support overall health and well-being.

5. **Balanced Macronutrients:** The diet promotes a balanced intake of

macronutrients, including proteins, healthy fats, and complex carbohydrates, focusing on the quality and sources of these nutrients.

6. **Stress Management and Lifestyle Factors:** Beyond just dietary aspects, the Galveston Diet encourages stress reduction techniques and lifestyle changes that support hormonal balance, such as adequate sleep, exercise, and mindfulness practices.

Benefits and Goals of Galveston Diet

Benefits of the Galveston Diet:

1. **Hormonal Balance:** The diet targets hormone regulation, especially insulin and cortisol, aiding in weight management and reducing symptoms related to hormonal fluctuations during menopause.

2. **Weight Management:** By focusing on hormone balance and anti-inflammatory foods, the diet assists in managing weight gain often associated with menopause, promoting a healthier body composition.

3. **Reduced Inflammation:** Emphasizing anti-inflammatory foods helps reduce inflammation within the body, potentially alleviating symptoms such as joint pain, bloating, and other discomforts related to inflammation.

4. **Improved Energy Levels:** The nutrient-dense foods and balanced macronutrients included in the diet can contribute to increased energy levels, supporting overall vitality and well-being.

5. **Enhanced Overall Health:** By promoting healthier eating habits and lifestyle changes, the Galveston Diet may contribute to improved health

markers, including heart health, blood sugar regulation, and overall well-being.

Goals of the Galveston Diet:

1. **Hormone Regulation:** The primary goal is to rebalance and regulate hormones, particularly insulin and cortisol, to manage weight and alleviate symptoms associated with hormonal changes during menopause.

2. **Weight Control:** The diet aims to help women maintain a healthy weight or manage weight gain commonly experienced during menopause.

3. **Inflammation Reduction:** By focusing on anti-inflammatory foods, the diet seeks to reduce inflammation, potentially easing discomfort caused by inflammatory processes in the body.

4. **Overall Wellness:** The diet strives to improve overall health, energy levels,

and well-being through healthy eating
habits and lifestyle adjustments.

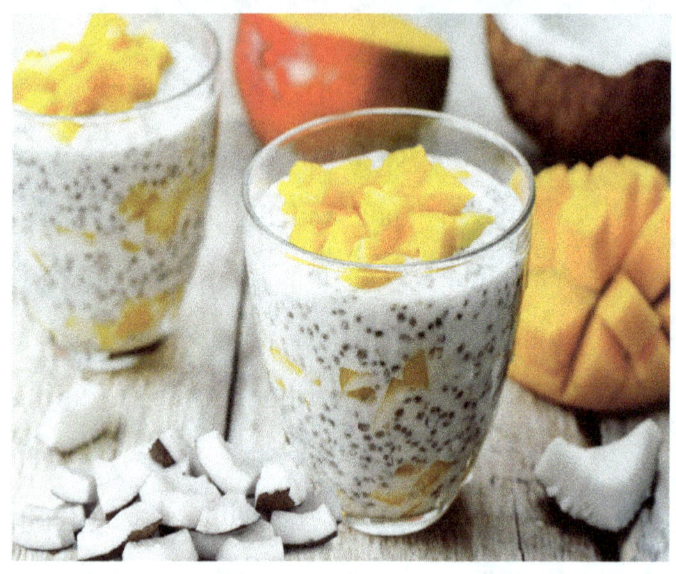

CHAPTER 2:

GETTING STARTED

Meal Planning and Preparation

1. **Understanding Dietary Guidelines:** Familiarize yourself with the Galveston Diet principles, focusing on hormone balance, anti-inflammatory foods, and nutrient-dense options.

2. **Create a Weekly Meal Plan:** Design a weekly meal plan incorporating the recommended foods and recipes aligned with the diet's guidelines. Consider a variety of options for breakfast, lunch, dinner, snacks, and beverages.

3. **Grocery Shopping:** Compile a shopping list based on the meal plan, ensuring you have all the necessary ingredients, especially focusing on fresh produce,

lean proteins, healthy fats, and anti-inflammatory foods.

4. **Preparation and Cooking:** Allocate time for food preparation, such as chopping vegetables, marinating proteins, and organizing ingredients for easy access during meal preparation.

5. **Batch Cooking and Portioning:** Consider batch cooking on weekends or free days to prepare meals in advance. Portion meals into appropriate serving sizes for easy access during the week.

6. **Mindful Cooking Practices:** Practice mindful cooking, focusing on healthy cooking methods like steaming, grilling, or baking. Use appropriate seasonings and avoid processed or unhealthy additives.

7. **Meal Timing and Intermittent Fasting:** Align meal times with intermittent fasting periods, especially

for overnight fasting, which is a key element of the Galveston Diet.

8. **Staying Consistent:** Maintain consistency with the meal plan and preparation, ensuring that the meals adhere to the Galveston Diet guidelines for hormone regulation and overall health improvement.

9. **Variety and Creativity:** Incorporate a diverse range of foods and recipes to maintain interest and enjoyment in the diet, ensuring a balance of nutrients and flavors.

Frequently Asked Questions (FAQs)

1. **What is the Galveston Diet?**

- The Galveston Diet is a specialized dietary approach designed for women experiencing menopause or perimenopause. It focuses on hormonal balance, weight management, and overall health during this phase.

2. **What are the key principles of the Galveston Diet?**

- The key principles include hormone regulation, anti-inflammatory foods, intermittent fasting, nutrient-dense eating, and lifestyle adjustments to support women during menopause.

3. **How does the diet help with menopausal symptoms?**

- By focusing on hormone regulation and reducing inflammation, the diet aims to alleviate symptoms commonly associated with menopause, such as weight gain, hot flashes, and mood swings.

4. **What foods are recommended on the Galveston Diet?**

- Recommended foods include vegetables, fruits, lean proteins, fatty fish, nuts, seeds, and healthy fats. Foods that reduce inflammation and support hormonal balance are emphasized.

5. Is intermittent fasting necessary for the Galveston Diet?

- Intermittent fasting, particularly overnight fasting, is a key component of the diet to regulate insulin levels and support the body's natural healing processes. However, its application can be personalized.

6. Can the diet be followed by individuals who are not in menopause?

- While specifically designed for menopausal women, the diet's focus on whole, nutrient-dense foods and anti-inflammatory options can benefit individuals of various life stages.

7. Are there specific exercise recommendations on the Galveston Diet?

- While exercise is not a primary focus, incorporating regular physical activity is beneficial for overall health. Recommendations often include a mix of cardiovascular and strength exercises.

8. **How quickly can one expect to see results on the Galveston Diet?**

- Results may vary, but some individuals notice changes in weight, energy levels, and symptom management within a few weeks to a couple of months of adhering to the diet.

9. **Are there support resources available for individuals following the Galveston Diet?**

- The Galveston Diet community often provides support through online resources, forums, recipes, and guidance to aid individuals in successfully following the diet.

10. **Is it essential to consult a healthcare provider before starting the Galveston Diet?**

- It's advisable to consult a healthcare professional before starting any new diet or lifestyle change, especially if you have existing health conditions or concerns.

Navigating Grocery Store

1. **Focus on Fresh Produce:** Prioritize the fresh produce section for a variety of vegetables and fruits. Choose colorful options rich in nutrients and antioxidants.

2. **Lean Proteins:** Head to the meat and seafood section for lean protein sources. Opt for skinless poultry, fish, and lean cuts of meat.

3. **Healthy Fats:** Look for healthy fats like avocados, nuts, seeds, and olive oil in the

aisles. These items are essential for the Galveston Diet.

4. **Whole Grains:** When selecting grains, prioritize whole grains like quinoa, brown rice, and whole wheat options. Check labels for whole grain content.

5. **Avoid Processed Foods:** Stay clear of processed and sugary items. Minimize packaged foods and those with added sugars or unhealthy additives.

6. **Read Labels:** Check food labels for hidden sugars, unhealthy fats, and additives. Look for products with minimal ingredients and without artificial additives.

7. **Anti-Inflammatory Foods:** Prioritize anti-inflammatory foods like leafy greens, berries, fatty fish, and turmeric. These foods can help reduce inflammation.

8. **Organic and Non-GMO Options:** Consider choosing organic or non-GMO options for produce, especially for items listed on the Dirty Dozen list, known for higher pesticide residues.

9. **Meal Preparation Staples:** Purchase items necessary for meal preparation, such as broth, spices, herbs, and vinegar for healthier cooking.

10. **Snack Wisely:** Look for healthier snack options like unsalted nuts, plain Greek yogurt, and fresh fruits for nutritious snacking.

11. **Plan Ahead:** Stick to your planned meals by shopping according to your pre-made meal plan to avoid purchasing unnecessary items.

12. Navigating the grocery store involves being mindful of food

One-week Grocery Shopping List

1. Fruits and Vegetables:

- Spinach

- Kale

- Broccoli

- Bell peppers (various colors)

- Berries (strawberries, blueberries)

- Avocados

- Lemons

2. Lean Proteins:

- Chicken breasts

- Salmon fillets

- Turkey breast slices

3. Healthy Fats:

- Almonds

- Chia seeds

- Olive oil

4. Whole Grains:

- Quinoa

- Brown rice

5. Dairy and Alternatives:

- Greek yogurt (plain, low-fat)
- Almond milk or coconut milk (unsweetened)

6. Anti-Inflammatory Foods:

- Turmeric
- Ginger

7. Herbs and Spices:

- Garlic
- Cinnamon
- Cumin
- Paprika

8. Other Essentials:

- Eggs
- Tofu (optional)
- Beans (black beans, chickpeas)
- Hummus
- Low-sodium vegetable broth
- Vinegar (apple cider or balsamic)
- Dark chocolate (70% or higher cocoa content)

9. **Snack Options:**

- Carrot sticks

- Hummus

- Greek yogurt with berries

- Nuts (almonds, walnuts)

10. **Beverages:**

- Green tea

- Sparkling water

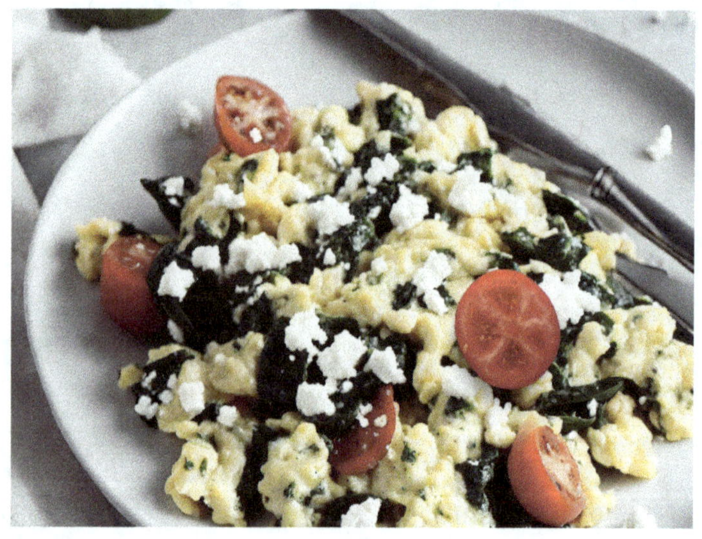

CHAPTER 3:

BREAKFAST INSPIRATIONS

Spinach and Feta Scramble

Ingredients:

- 2 eggs
- 1 cup fresh spinach
- 2 tablespoons crumbled feta cheese
- 1 tablespoon olive oil
- Salt and pepper to taste

Nutritional Information (Per Serving):

Calories	Protein	Fat	Carbohydrates
250	15g	18g	3g

Preparation Method:

1. Heat olive oil in a skillet over medium heat.
2. Add spinach and sauté until wilted.

3. Whisk eggs, pour into the skillet, and scramble with the spinach.

4. Add feta, season with salt and pepper, and cook until the eggs are set.

Coconut Chia Pudding

Ingredients:

- 1/4 cup chia seeds
- 1 cup coconut milk
- 1/2 teaspoon vanilla extract
- Berries or nuts for topping

Nutritional Information (Per Serving):

Calories	Protein	Fat	Carbohydrates
180	4g	12g	15g

Preparation Method:

1. Mix chia seeds, coconut milk, and vanilla extract in a bowl.

2. Refrigerate overnight or for at least 4 hours until it thickens.

3. Serve topped with berries or nuts.

Turkey and Veggie Breakfast Casserole

Ingredients:

- 8 eggs
- 1/2 cup diced bell peppers
- 1/2 cup diced onions
- 1 cup diced turkey sausage
- 1/2 cup shredded cheddar cheese
- Salt and pepper to taste

Nutritional Information (Per Serving):

Calories	Protein	Fat	Carbohydrates
280	22g	18g	6g

Preparation Method:

1. Preheat the oven to 350°F (175°C).

2. Whisk eggs and season with salt and pepper.

3. Grease a baking dish and layer the veggies, turkey sausage, and cheese.

4. Pour the whisked eggs over the mixture.

5. Bake for 25-30 minutes until set.

Avocado and Smoked Salmon Toast

Ingredients:

- 2 slices low-carb bread

- 1/2 avocado

- 2 slices smoked salmon

- Lemon juice

- Red pepper flakes (optional)

Nutritional Information (Per Serving):

Calories	Protein	Fat	Carbohydrates
300	18g	15g	20g

Preparation Method:

1. Toast the low-carb bread slices.

2. Mash avocado onto the toast, sprinkle with lemon juice.

3. Top with smoked salmon and red pepper flakes if desired.

Greek Yogurt Parfait

Ingredients:

- 1 cup Greek yogurt (unsweetened)
- 1/4 cup mixed berries (blueberries, raspberries)
- 2 tablespoons chopped nuts (almonds, walnuts)
- 1 teaspoon honey or a natural sweetener (optional)

Nutritional Information (Per Serving):

Calories	Protein	Fat	Carbohydrates
220	20g	10g	15g

Preparation Method:

1. In a glass, layer Greek yogurt, berries, and nuts.
2. Drizzle with honey for sweetness if desired.

Low-Carb Breakfast Burrito

Ingredients:

- 2 large lettuce leaves
- 2 eggs
- 1/4 cup diced tomatoes
- 1/4 cup diced bell peppers
- 2 slices turkey bacon, cooked
- Salt, pepper, and cumin to taste

Nutritional Information (Per Serving):

Calories	Protein	Fat	Carbohydrates
280	18g	15g	8g

Preparation Method:

1. Heat a non-stick skillet over medium heat.
2. Scramble the eggs, adding tomatoes and bell peppers.
3. Season with salt, pepper, and cumin.
4. Lay out lettuce leaves, place the egg mixture and turkey bacon, then roll them up.

Almond Flour Pancakes

Ingredients:

- 1 cup almond flour
- 2 eggs
- 1/4 cup unsweetened almond milk
- 1/2 teaspoon baking powder
- 1 teaspoon vanilla extract

Nutritional Information (Per Serving):

Calories	Protein	Fat	Carbohydrates
280	12g	22g	8g

Preparation Method:

1. Mix almond flour, eggs, almond milk, baking powder, and vanilla extract.
2. Cook pancake batter on a non-stick skillet over medium heat until golden on each side.

Veggie Omelette Cups

Ingredients:

- 6 eggs
- 1/2 cup diced bell peppers
- 1/2 cup diced spinach
- 1/4 cup diced onions
- 1/4 cup shredded cheese
- Salt and pepper to taste

Nutritional Information (Per Serving - 2 cups):

Calories	Protein	Fat	Carbohydrates

220	16g	15g	6g

Preparation Method:

1. Preheat the oven to 350°F (175°C).

2. Grease a muffin tin.

3. Whisk eggs, mix in veggies, cheese, salt, and pepper.

4. Pour the mixture evenly into the muffin tin.

5. Bake for 20-25 minutes until eggs are set.

Protein-Packed Breakfast Bowl

Ingredients:

- 1/2 cup quinoa, cooked
- 1/4 cup black beans, drained and rinsed
- 2 tablespoons diced avocado
- 2 tablespoons salsa
- 2 tablespoons plain Greek yogurt
- Cilantro for garnish

- Lime wedges (optional)

Nutritional Information (Per Serving):

Calories	Protein	Fat	Carbohydrates
300	15g	10g	35g

Preparation Method:

1. In a bowl, layer cooked quinoa, black beans, avocado, salsa, and Greek yogurt.
2. Garnish with cilantro and serve with lime wedges if desired.

Zucchini and Egg Muffins

Ingredients:

- 4 eggs
- 1 cup grated zucchini
- 1/4 cup diced onions
- 1/4 cup diced bell peppers
- 1/4 cup grated cheese
- Salt, pepper, and garlic powder to taste

Nutritional Information (Per Serving - 2 muffins):

Calories	Protein	Fat	Carbohydrates
200	14g	12g	8g

Preparation Method:

1. Preheat the oven to 350°F (175°C).
2. Whisk eggs and mix in grated zucchini, onions, bell peppers, cheese, salt, pepper, and garlic powder.
3. Pour the mixture into a greased muffin tin.
4. Bake for 20-25 minutes until set.

Egg and Veggie Wrap

Ingredients:

- 2 large whole wheat or low-carb tortillas
- 4 eggs, scrambled

- 1/2 cup sautéed mixed veggies (bell peppers, onions, spinach)
- 1/4 cup shredded cheese
- Salsa or hot sauce (optional)

Nutritional Information (Per Serving):

Calories	Protein	Fat	Carbohydrates
320	20g	15g	25g

Preparation Method:

1. Lay out tortillas and fill them with scrambled eggs, sautéed veggies, and shredded cheese.
2. Roll up the tortillas and, if desired, warm them in a pan to melt the cheese.
3. Serve with salsa or hot sauce if preferred.

Cottage Cheese and Berry Bowl

Ingredients:

- 1 cup low-fat cottage cheese

- 1/2 cup mixed berries (strawberries, blueberries)
- 2 tablespoons chopped nuts (almonds, walnuts)
- 1 teaspoon honey (optional)

Nutritional Information (Per Serving):

Calories	Protein	Fat	Carbohydrates
250	25g	10g	15g

Preparation Method:

1. In a bowl, combine cottage cheese, mixed berries, and chopped nuts.
2. Drizzle with honey for added sweetness, if desired.

Sweet Potato and Egg Hash

Ingredients:

- 1 medium sweet potato, diced
- 2 eggs

- 1/4 cup diced red bell peppers
- 1/4 cup diced red onions
- 1 tablespoon olive oil
- Salt, pepper, and paprika to taste

Nutritional Information (Per Serving):

Calories	Protein	Fat	Carbohydrates
280	10g	10g	35g

Preparation Method:

1. Heat olive oil in a skillet over medium heat.
2. Add sweet potatoes and cook until slightly browned and softened.
3. Add bell peppers and onions, continue cooking until veggies are tender.
4. Push the veggies to the side, crack eggs into the skillet, and scramble until cooked.

5. Season with salt, pepper, and paprika before serving.

Low-Carb Eggplant and Tomato Stacks

Ingredients:

- 1 large eggplant, sliced
- 2 tomatoes, sliced
- 1/4 cup shredded mozzarella cheese
- Fresh basil leaves
- Olive oil
- Salt and pepper to taste

Nutritional Information (Per Serving - 2 stacks):

Calories	Protein	Fat	Carbohydrates
220	8g	12g	15g

Preparation Method:

1. Preheat the oven to 375°F (190°C).

2. Brush eggplant slices with olive oil and season with salt and pepper. Roast for 10-15 minutes until tender.

3. Layer roasted eggplant, tomato slices, mozzarella, and basil leaves to create stacks.

4. Place back in the oven for a few minutes until the cheese melts.

Mushroom and Spinach Frittata

Ingredients:

- 6 eggs
- 1 cup sliced mushrooms
- 2 cups fresh spinach
- 1/4 cup grated Parmesan cheese
- 1 tablespoon olive oil
- Salt and pepper to taste

Nutritional Information (Per Serving - 2 slices):

Calories	Protein	Fat	Carbohydrates
260	18g	18g	5g

Preparation Method:

1. Preheat oven to 350°F (175°C).

2. In an oven-safe skillet, sauté mushrooms and spinach in olive oil until wilted.

3. Whisk eggs, add to the skillet, and cook for a few minutes until the edges set.

4. Sprinkle with Parmesan cheese and transfer to the oven. Bake until fully set.

Low-Carb Breakfast Sausage Wraps

Ingredients:

- 4 turkey or chicken sausage patties
- 4 large lettuce leaves
- 1/4 cup diced tomatoes
- 1/4 cup diced onions
- Mustard or hot sauce (optional)

Nutritional Information (Per Serving - 2 wraps):

Calories	Protein	Fat	Carbohydrates
220	18g	12g	10g

Preparation Method:

1. Cook sausage patties according to package instructions.
2. Lay out lettuce leaves, place sausage, tomatoes, onions, and add condiments if desired.
3. Roll up the lettuce leaves and serve.

Savory Cauliflower Rice Breakfast Bowl

Ingredients:

- 1 cup cauliflower rice
- 2 eggs
- 1/4 cup diced bell peppers
- 1/4 cup diced turkey bacon or chicken sausage

- 1 tablespoon olive oil
- Salt, pepper, and herbs of choice

Nutritional Information (Per Serving):

Calories	Protein	Fat	Carbohydrates
270	15g	18g	10g

Preparation Method:

1. In a skillet, heat olive oil over medium heat.
2. Add cauliflower rice, bell peppers, and protein (bacon or sausage). Sauté until cauliflower is tender.
3. Create space in the pan, crack eggs, and scramble until cooked through.
4. Season with salt, pepper, and preferred herbs before serving.

Low-Carb Breakfast Pizza

Ingredients:

- 1 low-carb tortilla or flatbread

- 2 tablespoons tomato sauce or marinara

- 1/4 cup shredded mozzarella cheese

- 2 slices turkey or chicken bacon, chopped

- 1 egg

- Fresh basil or arugula for topping

Nutritional Information (Per Serving):

Calories	Protein	Fat	Carbohydrates
290	18g	15g	15g

Preparation Method:

1. Preheat the oven to 375°F (190°C).

2. Place the tortilla on a baking sheet and spread tomato sauce over it.

3. Sprinkle with mozzarella cheese, add chopped bacon, and create a well in the center for the egg.

4. Crack the egg into the well and bake for 10-15 minutes or until the egg is cooked to your preference.

5. Top with fresh herbs before serving.

Spinach and Mushroom Breakfast Quesadilla

Ingredients:

- 2 low-carb or whole wheat tortillas
- 1/2 cup cooked spinach
- 1/2 cup sautéed mushrooms
- 1/4 cup shredded cheddar or Mexican blend cheese
- 1 tablespoon olive oil
- Salsa or Greek yogurt for dipping (optional)

Nutritional Information (Per Serving):

Calories	Protein	Fat	Carbohydrates
310	14g	18g	25g

Preparation Method:

1. Heat a skillet over medium heat with olive oil.

2. Place one tortilla in the skillet and top with cooked spinach, mushrooms, and cheese.

3. Place the second tortilla on top, press down gently, and cook until both sides are crispy and cheese is melted.

4. Slice into wedges and serve with salsa or Greek yogurt for dipping.

Low-Carb Breakfast Quiche Cups

Ingredients:

- 4 eggs
- 1/4 cup diced bell peppers
- 1/4 cup diced onions
- 1/4 cup diced ham or turkey
- 1/4 cup shredded mozzarella cheese
- Salt, pepper, and herbs of choice

Nutritional Information (Per Serving - 2 cups):

Calories	Protein	Fat	Carbohydrates
250	18g	15g	8g

Preparation Method:

1. Preheat oven to 350°F (175°C).
2. In a bowl, whisk eggs, then mix in bell peppers, onions, protein, cheese, salt, and pepper.
3. Pour the mixture evenly into a greased muffin tin.
4. Bake for 20-25 minutes until set.

Low-Carb Breakfast Sausage Skillet

Ingredients:

- 4 turkey or chicken sausage links, sliced
- 1 cup cauliflower florets
- 1/2 cup sliced zucchini

- 1/4 cup diced onions

- 2 eggs

- 2 tablespoons olive oil

- Salt, pepper, and smoked paprika to taste

Nutritional Information (Per Serving):

Calories	Protein	Fat	Carbohydrates
290	16g	20g	8g

Preparation Method:

1. Heat olive oil in a skillet over medium heat.

2. Sauté sausage slices until browned, then add cauliflower, zucchini, and onions.

3. Cook until the veggies are tender. Season with salt, pepper, and smoked paprika.

4. Create wells in the skillet, crack eggs, and cook until desired doneness.

Mediterranean Breakfast Stuffed Peppers

Ingredients:

- 2 large bell peppers
- 4 eggs
- 1/2 cup diced tomatoes
- 1/4 cup crumbled feta cheese
- Fresh parsley for garnish
- Olive oil
- Salt and pepper to taste

Nutritional Information (Per Serving - 1 pepper):

Calories	Protein	Fat	Carbohydrates
260	15g	14g	15g

Preparation Method:

1. Preheat the oven to 375°F (190°C).
2. Cut the tops off the bell peppers, remove seeds, and place them in a baking dish.

3. Divide diced tomatoes and feta cheese into the peppers.

4. Crack an egg into each pepper, season with salt and pepper, and bake for 20-25 minutes.

5. Garnish with fresh parsley before serving.

Broccoli and Cheddar Egg Muffins

Ingredients:

- 6 eggs
- 1 cup chopped broccoli florets
- 1/4 cup shredded cheddar cheese
- 1/4 cup diced red bell peppers
- 1 tablespoon olive oil
- Salt, pepper, and garlic powder to taste

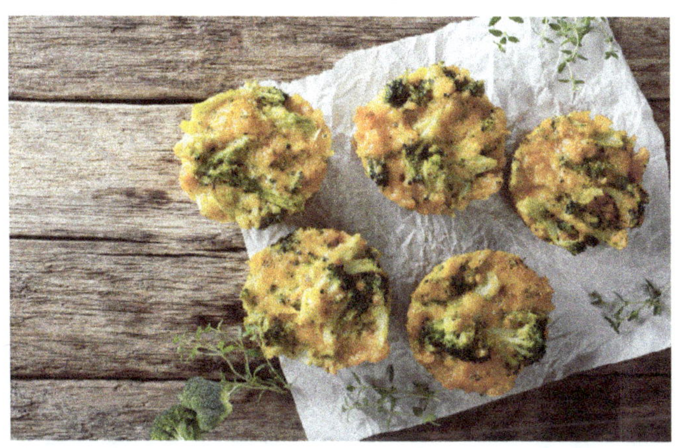

Nutritional Information (Per Serving - 2 muffins):

Calories	Protein	Fat	Carbohydrates
280	18g	20g	6g

Preparation Method:

1. Preheat the oven to 350°F (175°C).

2. In a skillet, sauté broccoli and bell peppers in olive oil until slightly tender.

3. Whisk eggs and mix in sautéed veggies, cheese, salt, pepper, and garlic powder.

4. Pour the mixture evenly into a greased muffin tin.

5. Bake for 20-25 minutes until set.

Low-Carb Breakfast Tacos

Ingredients:

- 4 small low-carb tortillas
- 1/2 cup black beans, drained and rinsed
- 4 eggs, scrambled
- 1/4 cup diced avocado
- Salsa or hot sauce (optional)

Nutritional Information (Per Serving - 2 tacos):

Calories	Protein	Fat	Carbohydrates
300	18g	15g	20g

Preparation Method:

1. Warm tortillas in a skillet or microwave.
2. Divide black beans and scrambled eggs among the tortillas.

3. Top with diced avocado and salsa or hot
    sauce if desired.

59

CHAPTER 4:

SATISFYING LUNCH CREATIONS

Grilled Chicken Salad

Ingredients:

- Grilled chicken breast
- Mixed greens (spinach, arugula)
- Cherry tomatoes
- Cucumber slices
- Red onion
- Olive oil and balsamic vinegar for dressing

Nutritional Information (Per Serving):

Calories	Protein	Fat	Carbohydrates
350	25g	12g	15g

Preparation Method:

1. Grill the chicken breast and slice it.

2. Assemble a salad with mixed greens, cherry tomatoes, cucumber slices, red onion, and grilled chicken.

3. Drizzle with olive oil and balsamic vinegar for dressing.

Salmon and Asparagus Foil Packets

Ingredients:

- Salmon filet
- Asparagus spears
- Lemon slices
- Olive oil
- Garlic, salt, and pepper

Nutritional Information (Per Serving):

Calories	Protein	Fat	Carbohydrates
400	30g	20g	10g

Preparation Method:

1. Place a salmon filet and asparagus spears on a sheet of foil.

2. Drizzle with olive oil, add garlic, lemon slices, salt, and pepper.

3. Seal the foil and bake in the oven for 15-20 minutes.

Turkey Lettuce Wraps

Ingredients:

- Turkey breast slices
- Lettuce leaves
- Avocado slices
- Tomato, thinly sliced
- Mustard or hummus (optional)

Nutritional Information (Per Serving):

Calories	Protein	Fat	Carbohydrates
300	20g	10g	10g

Preparation Method:

1. Lay out lettuce leaves and fill with turkey slices, avocado, tomato, and optional condiments like mustard or hummus.

2. Roll up the lettuce to form wraps.

Quinoa and Black Bean Stuffed Bell Peppers

Ingredients:

- Bell peppers
- Cooked quinoa
- Black beans
- Diced tomatoes
- Onion, chopped
- Shredded cheese (optional)
- Olive oil, cumin, paprika, salt, and pepper

Nutritional Information (Per Serving):

Calories	Protein	Fat	Carbohydrates

350	12g	8g	45g	

Preparation Method:

1. Cut the tops off the bell peppers and remove seeds.

2. In a bowl, mix cooked quinoa, black beans, diced tomatoes, chopped onion, and seasoning.

3. Stuff the bell peppers with the mixture and bake for 25-30 minutes. Top with cheese if desired.

Egg Salad Lettuce Wraps

Ingredients:

- Hard-boiled eggs, chopped
- Greek yogurt or mayonnaise
- Diced celery
- Dijon mustard
- Lettuce leaves for wrapping

Nutritional Information (Per Serving):

Calories	Protein	Fat	Carbohydrates
250	12g	15g	5g

Preparation Method:

1. In a bowl, combine chopped hard-boiled eggs, Greek yogurt or mayonnaise, diced celery, and Dijon mustard.

2. Scoop the egg salad into lettuce leaves and wrap them up.

Tuna and Avocado Salad

Ingredients:

- Canned tuna in water
- Avocado, diced
- Diced red onion
- Chopped cilantro
- Lime juice
- Salt and pepper

Nutritional Information (Per Serving):

Calories	Protein	Fat	Carbohydrates
320	25g	15g	10g

Preparation Method:

1. In a bowl, mix tuna, diced avocado, red onion, cilantro, lime juice, salt, and pepper.
2. Serve the tuna salad on its own or over a bed of greens.

Mediterranean Chickpea Salad

Ingredients:

- Canned chickpeas, drained
- Chopped cucumber
- Diced tomatoes
- Chopped red bell pepper
- Kalamata olives
- Feta cheese (optional)

- Olive oil, red wine vinegar, oregano, salt, and pepper

Nutritional Information (Per Serving):

Calories	Protein	Fat	Carbohydrates
280	10g	12g	30g

Preparation Method:

1. In a bowl, combine chickpeas, cucumber, tomatoes, bell pepper, and olives.
2. Toss with olive oil, red wine vinegar, oregano, salt, and pepper. Add feta cheese if desired.

Stir-Fried Tofu and Vegetable Quinoa Bowl

Ingredients:

- Firm tofu, cubed
- Quinoa, cooked

- Mixed vegetables (bell peppers, broccoli, carrots)

- Soy sauce or tamari

- Sesame oil

- Garlic, minced

- Green onions for garnish

Nutritional Information (Per Serving):

Calories	Protein	Fat	Carbohydrates
350	18g	12g	35g

Preparation Method:

1. In a skillet, stir-fry tofu and mixed vegetables with sesame oil and minced garlic.

2. Add cooked quinoa, soy sauce or tamari for seasoning, and cook until heated through.

3. Serve in a bowl, garnished with green onions.

Chicken and Vegetable Lettuce Wraps

Ingredients:

- Grilled chicken strips
- Sliced bell peppers
- Sliced carrots
- Sliced cucumber
- Lettuce leaves for wrapping
- Tahini or peanut sauce for dipping (optional)

Nutritional Information (Per Serving):

Calories	Protein	Fat	Carbohydrates
250	20g	10g	15g

Preparation Method:

1. Arrange grilled chicken strips, bell peppers, carrots, and cucumber on lettuce leaves.

2. Roll the ingredients in the lettuce leaves and serve with tahini or peanut sauce if desired.

Shrimp and Quinoa Salad

Ingredients:

- Cooked shrimp
- Cooked quinoa
- Diced avocado
- Diced red onion
- Chopped cilantro
- Lime juice
- Olive oil, salt, and pepper

Nutritional Information (Per Serving):

Calories	Protein	Fat	Carbohydrates
280	20g	10g	25g

Preparation Method:

1. Combine cooked shrimp, quinoa, diced avocado, red onion, and cilantro in a bowl.

2. Dress with lime juice, olive oil, salt, and pepper.

Turkey and Hummus Wrap

Ingredients:

- Sliced turkey breast
- Whole wheat or low-carb wrap
- Hummus
- Shredded lettuce
- Thinly sliced red bell peppers
- Sliced pickles

Nutritional Information(Per Serving):

Calories	Protein	Fat	Carbohydrates
320	20g	10g	30g

Preparation Method:

1. Spread hummus on the wrap.

2. Layer the wrap with turkey slices, shredded lettuce, sliced bell peppers, and pickles.

3. Roll up the wrap and slice in half.

Eggplant and Zucchini Ratatouille

Ingredients:

- Eggplant, diced
- Zucchini, diced
- Diced tomatoes
- Chopped onions
- Minced garlic
- Olive oil, thyme, basil, salt, and pepper

Nutritional Information (Per Serving):

Calories	Protein	Fat	Carbohydrates
300	8g	10g	30g

Preparation Method:

1. In a skillet, sauté onions and garlic in olive oil until soft.

2. Add diced eggplant, zucchini, and tomatoes. Season with thyme, basil, salt, and pepper.

3. Simmer until the vegetables are tender.

Greek Chicken Bowls

Ingredients:

- Grilled chicken breast, sliced

- Cooked quinoa or brown rice

- Diced cucumbers

- Cherry tomatoes, halved

- Red onion, thinly sliced

- Kalamata olives

- Feta cheese

- Greek dressing (olive oil, lemon juice, oregano)

Nutritional Information (Per Serving):

Calories	Protein	Fat	Carbohydrates
350	25g	12g	25g

Preparation Method:

1. Arrange grilled chicken, quinoa or brown rice, cucumbers, tomatoes, red onion, and olives in a bowl.

2. Sprinkle with feta cheese and drizzle with Greek dressing.

Tofu Stir-Fry with Broccoli and Cashews

Ingredients:

- Firm tofu, cubed
- Broccoli florets
- Cashews
- Soy sauce or tamari
- Sesame oil
- Minced garlic and ginger
- Green onions for garnish

Nutritional Information (Per Serving):

Calories	Protein	Fat	Carbohydrates
320	20g	15g	20g

Preparation Method:

1. Stir-fry cubed tofu in sesame oil until lightly browned. Set aside.

2. In the same pan, stir-fry broccoli, cashews, garlic, and ginger until the broccoli is tender.

3. Add the tofu back to the pan, season with soy sauce or tamari, and cook until heated through.

4. Garnish with green onions before serving.

Mediterranean Lentil Salad

Ingredients:

- Cooked lentils
- Chopped cucumbers

- Diced red bell pepper

- Chopped parsley

- Red onion, finely diced

- Lemon juice and olive oil

- Cumin, salt, and pepper

Nutritional Information (Per Serving):

Calories	Protein	Fat	Carbohydrates
250	15g	8g	35g

Preparation Method:

1. Combine cooked lentils, cucumbers, red bell pepper, parsley, and red onion in a bowl.

2. Dress with lemon juice, olive oil, and season with cumin, salt, and pepper.

Turkey Lettuce Cups with Mango Salsa

Ingredients:

- Ground turkey

- Lettuce leaves
- Diced mango
- Diced red onion
- Chopped cilantro
- Lime juice
- Chili powder, salt, and pepper

Nutritional Information (Per Serving):

Calories	Protein	Fat	Carbohydrates
320	20g	12g	20g

Preparation Method:

1. Cook ground turkey with chili powder, salt, and pepper until fully cooked.

2. In a separate bowl, mix diced mango, red onion, cilantro, and lime juice to make salsa.

3. Spoon the turkey into lettuce leaves and top with mango salsa.

Salmon and Avocado Nori Rolls

Ingredients:

- Nori seaweed sheets
- Cooked and flaked salmon
- Sliced avocado
- Shredded carrots
- Cucumber matchsticks
- Wasabi (optional)
- Soy sauce or tamari for dipping

Nutritional Information (Per Serving):

Calories	Protein	Fat	Carbohydrates
350	25g	18g	10g

Preparation Method:

1. Lay out a nori sheet and spread flaked salmon along one edge.
2. Add avocado slices, shredded carrots, and cucumber matchsticks.

3. Roll up the nori sheet tightly. Slice into pieces and serve with soy sauce and optional wasabi.

Mushroom and Spinach Quiche

Ingredients:

- Pie crust (whole wheat or low-carb)
- Eggs
- Sliced mushrooms
- Chopped spinach
- Diced onions
- Shredded cheese
- Milk or almond milk
- Garlic powder, salt, and pepper

Nutritional Information (Per Serving):

Calories	Protein	Fat	Carbohydrates
300	12g	15g	20g

Preparation Method:

1. Preheat the oven to 375°F (190°C).

2. Line a pie dish with the crust.

3. Sauté mushrooms, spinach, and onions until tender.

4. Whisk together eggs, milk, shredded cheese, garlic powder, salt, and pepper.

5. Pour the egg mixture over the sautéed vegetables in the pie crust.

6. Bake for 30-35 minutes or until the quiche is set.

Cauliflower Fried "Rice" with Shrimp

Ingredients:

- Cauliflower rice
- Shrimp, peeled and deveined
- Mixed vegetables (peas, carrots, bell peppers)
- Minced ginger and garlic
- Soy sauce or tamari
- Scrambled eggs (optional)
- Sesame oil

Nutritional Information (Per Serving):

Calories	Protein	Fat	Carbohydrates
320	22g	12g	20g

Preparation Method:

1. Stir-fry shrimp in sesame oil until cooked. Set aside.
2. In the same pan, stir-fry mixed vegetables, ginger, and garlic.
3. Add cauliflower rice and soy sauce. Cook until heated through.
4. Add the cooked shrimp back to the pan and scramble in eggs if desired.

Zoodle (Zucchini Noodle) Pasta with Turkey Meatballs

Ingredients:

- Zucchini noodles (zoodles)
- Ground turkey

- Marinara sauce (low-sugar)

- Italian seasoning, salt, and pepper

- Olive oil

- Grated Parmesan cheese (optional)

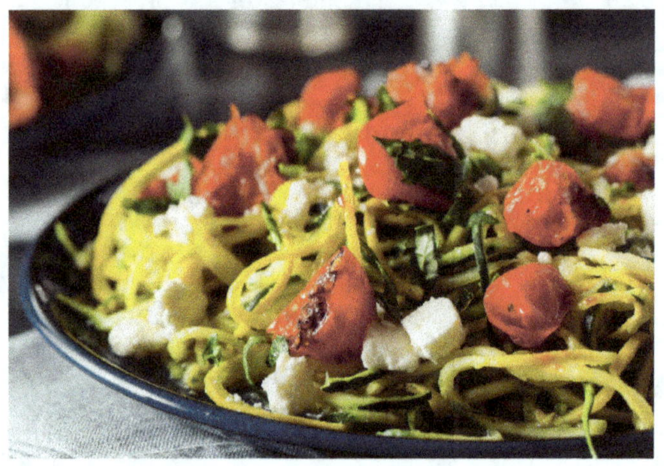

Nutritional Information (Per Serving):

Calories	Protein	Fat	Carbohydrates
350	25g	15g	20g

Preparation Method:

1. Form ground turkey into meatballs and bake in the oven.

2. In a pan, sauté zucchini noodles in olive oil until slightly softened.

3. Heat the marinara sauce and add the cooked meatballs.

4. Serve the meatballs and sauce over the zucchini noodles. Sprinkle with Parmesan cheese if desired.

Mediterranean Chicken Wrap

Ingredients:

- Grilled chicken strips
- Whole wheat or low-carb wrap
- Tzatziki sauce
- Sliced cucumber
- Diced tomatoes
- Red onion slices
- Fresh spinach

Nutritional Information (Per Serving):

Calories	Protein	Fat	Carbohydrates

300	25g	10g	30g

Preparation Method:

1. Lay out the wrap and spread tzatziki sauce.
2. Add grilled chicken, cucumber slices, tomatoes, red onion, and fresh spinach.
3. Roll up the wrap and slice in half.

Black Bean and Corn Salad

Ingredients:

- Canned black beans, drained and rinsed
- Corn kernels (fresh or thawed if frozen)
- Diced bell peppers (various colors)
- Chopped cilantro
- Lime juice
- Olive oil, cumin, salt, and pepper

Nutritional Information (Per Serving):

Calories	Protein	Fat	Carbohydrates

250	10g	8g	35g

Preparation Method:

1. In a bowl, combine black beans, corn, bell peppers, and cilantro.

2. Dress with lime juice, olive oil, cumin, salt, and pepper.

Turkey and Hummus Plate

Ingredients:

- Sliced turkey breast
- Hummus
- Sliced cucumber
- Cherry tomatoes
- Sliced bell peppers
- Whole grain crackers or pita bread

Nutritional Information (Per Serving):

Calories	Protein	Fat	Carbohydrates

| 280 | 20g | 10g | 25g |

Preparation Method:

1. Arrange sliced turkey, hummus, cucumber, tomatoes, and bell peppers on a plate.
2. Serve with whole grain crackers or pita bread.

Caprese Salad with Grilled Chicken

Ingredients:

- Grilled chicken breast, sliced
- Sliced fresh mozzarella
- Sliced tomatoes
- Fresh basil leaves
- Balsamic glaze
- Olive oil, salt, and pepper

Nutritional Information (Per Serving):

Calories	Protein	Fat	Carbohydrates

350	30g	15g	10g

Preparation Method:

1. Arrange sliced grilled chicken, fresh mozzarella, and tomato slices on a plate.

2. Top with fresh basil leaves, drizzle with balsamic glaze, and a dash of olive oil. Season with salt and pepper.

CHAPTER 5:

DINNER DELICACIES

Grilled Lemon Herb Chicken

Ingredients:

- Chicken breast
- Lemon juice
- Fresh herbs (thyme, rosemary)
- Garlic, minced
- Olive oil
- Salt and pepper

Nutritional Information(Per Serving):

Calories	Protein	Fat	Carbohydrates
300	25g	10g	5g

Preparation Method:

1. Marinate chicken in lemon juice, herbs, garlic, olive oil, salt, and pepper.

2. Grill until cooked through and serve with a side of roasted vegetables or a green salad.

Baked Salmon with Dill Sauce

Ingredients:

- Salmon filets
- Fresh dill
- Greek yogurt
- Lemon zest
- Dijon mustard
- Garlic powder, salt, and pepper

Nutritional Information (Per Serving):

Calories	Protein	Fat	Carbohydrates
300	25g	15g	10g

Preparation Method:

1. Season salmon with salt, pepper, and lemon zest.

2. Bake until flaky. For the sauce, mix Greek yogurt, dill, Dijon mustard, garlic powder, and serve over the salmon.

Zucchini Noodles with Pesto and Grilled Shrimp

Ingredients:

- Zucchini noodles (zoodles)
- Shrimp, peeled and deveined
- Pesto sauce
- Olive oil
- Cherry tomatoes
- Pine nuts (optional)

Nutritional Information (Per Serving):

Calories	Protein	Fat	Carbohydrates
280	20g	12g	15g

Preparation Method:

1. Sauté shrimp in olive oil until cooked, set aside.

2. In the same pan, sauté zucchini noodles until tender.

3. Toss zoodles with pesto, top with grilled shrimp, cherry tomatoes, and pine nuts if desired.

Taco Stuffed Bell Peppers

Ingredients:

- Bell peppers
- Ground turkey or beef
- Taco seasoning
- Black beans
- Diced tomatoes
- Shredded cheese (optional)

Nutritional Information (Per Serving):

Calories	Protein	Fat	Carbohydrates
350	25g	15g	20g

Preparation Method:

1. Cut bell peppers in half, removing seeds and membranes.

2. Cook ground meat with taco seasoning, then mix in black beans and diced tomatoes.

3. Fill bell peppers with the meat mixture, top with cheese if desired, and bake until peppers are tender.

Mediterranean Grilled Veggie Skewers

Ingredients:

- Assorted vegetables (bell peppers, zucchini, cherry tomatoes, red onion)
- Olive oil
- Balsamic vinegar
- Garlic, minced
- Italian seasoning, salt, and pepper

Nutritional Information (Per Serving):

Calories	Protein	Fat	Carbohydrates
250	5g	10g	25g

Preparation Method:

1. Cut vegetables into chunks and thread onto skewers.

2. Whisk together olive oil, balsamic vinegar, minced garlic, Italian seasoning, salt, and pepper for the marinade.

3. Brush the marinade over the skewered vegetables and grill until tender.

Cauliflower Crust Pizza

Ingredients:

- Cauliflower, grated and cooked
- Eggs
- Mozzarella cheese
- Pizza sauce (low-sugar)
- Toppings: bell peppers, onions, mushrooms, spinach

- Italian seasoning

Nutritional Information(Per Serving):

Calories	Protein	Fat	Carbohydrates
300	15g	10g	20g

Preparation Method:

1. Mix cooked cauliflower, eggs, and mozzarella cheese to form a dough.
2. Press the dough into a pizza shape and bake until golden.
3. Top with sauce, veggies, and cheese. Bake until toppings are cooked.

Stir-Fried Tofu and Broccoli

Ingredients:

- Firm tofu, cubed
- Broccoli florets
- Bell peppers, sliced
- Soy sauce or tamari

- Sesame oil

- Minced ginger and garlic

- Green onions for garnish

Nutritional Information (Per Serving):

Calories	Protein	Fat	Carbohydrates
320	20g	12g	15g

Preparation Method:

1. Stir-fry tofu until golden. Set aside.

2. Stir-fry broccoli, bell peppers, ginger, and garlic in sesame oil until crisp-tender.

3. Add the tofu back to the pan, season with soy sauce, and cook until heated through.

4. Garnish with green onions before serving.

Lemon Herb Quinoa with Grilled Chicken

Ingredients:

- Quinoa, cooked

- Grilled chicken breast, sliced

- Lemon juice

- Fresh herbs (parsley, thyme)

- Olive oil

- Salt and pepper

Nutritional Information (Per Serving):

Calories	Protein	Fat	Carbohydrates
300	25g	10g	25g

Preparation Method:

1. Toss cooked quinoa with lemon juice, herbs, olive oil, salt, and pepper.

2. Serve with grilled chicken slices on top.

Garlic Shrimp with Quinoa and Roasted Vegetables

Ingredients:

- Shrimp, peeled and deveined

- Quinoa, cooked
- Assorted vegetables (such as bell peppers, asparagus, and cherry tomatoes)
- Garlic, minced
- Olive oil
- Lemon zest
- Salt and pepper

Nutritional Information (Per Serving):

Calories	Protein	Fat	Carbohydrates
350	25g	10g	30g

Preparation Method:

1. Toss shrimp with minced garlic, lemon zest, olive oil, salt, and pepper.
2. Roast vegetables in the oven until tender.
3. Sauté the seasoned shrimp until cooked.
4. Serve shrimp and roasted vegetables over a bed of cooked quinoa.

Spaghetti Squash with Turkey Bolognese

Ingredients:

- Spaghetti squash
- Ground turkey
- Tomato sauce (low-sugar)
- Onion, diced
- Garlic, minced
- Italian seasoning, salt, and pepper

Nutritional Information (Per Serving):

Calories	Protein	Fat	Carbohydrates
300	20g	10g	20g

Preparation Method:

1. Roast spaghetti squash until tender and scrape out the "noodles."
2. Sauté ground turkey with onions and garlic until browned.

3. Add tomato sauce, Italian seasoning, salt, and pepper. Simmer for 15-20 minutes.

4. Serve the turkey Bolognese over the spaghetti squash.

Lemon Herb Baked Cod

Ingredients:

- Cod filets
- Lemon juice
- Fresh herbs (such as dill, parsley)
- Garlic powder
- Olive oil
- Salt and pepper

Nutritional Information (Per Serving):

Calories	Protein	Fat	Carbohydrates
250	30g	10g	5g

Preparation Method:

1. Place cod fillets in a baking dish.

2. Mix lemon juice, herbs, garlic powder, olive oil, salt, and pepper.

3. Pour the mixture over the fish and bake until the fish is cooked through.

Beef and Vegetable Stir-Fry

Ingredients:

- Beef strips
- Mixed vegetables (such as broccoli, bell peppers, snap peas)
- Soy sauce or tamari
- Sesame oil
- Minced ginger and garlic
- Green onions for garnish

Nutritional Information (Per Serving):

Calories	Protein	Fat	Carbohydrates
350	25g	15g	20g

Preparation Method:

1. Stir-fry beef strips until browned. Set aside.

2. Stir-fry mixed vegetables, ginger, and garlic in sesame oil.

3. Add the beef back to the pan, season with soy sauce, and cook until heated through.

4. Garnish with green onions before serving.

Lemon Garlic Chicken with Steamed Broccoli

Ingredients:

- Chicken thighs or breasts
- Lemon juice
- Minced garlic
- Olive oil
- Italian seasoning
- Salt and pepper
- Broccoli florets

Nutritional Information (Per Serving):

Calories	Protein	Fat	Carbohydrates
350	25g	15g	10g

Preparation Method:

1. Marinate chicken in lemon juice, minced garlic, olive oil, Italian seasoning, salt, and pepper.
2. Bake or grill until cooked through.
3. Steam broccoli and serve as a side.

Blackened Mahi-Mahi with Avocado Salsa

Ingredients:

- Mahi-Mahi filets
- Blackening seasoning (paprika, cumin, cayenne, garlic powder)
- Avocado, diced
- Red onion, finely chopped
- Cilantro, chopped

- Lime juice

- Olive oil

- Salt and pepper

Nutritional Information (Per Serving):

Calories	Protein	Fat	Carbohydrates
300	30g	15g	10g

Preparation Method:

1. Coat Mahi-Mahi with blackening seasoning and grill or bake until cooked.

2. Mix diced avocado, red onion, cilantro, lime juice, olive oil, salt, and pepper for the salsa.

3. Serve the fish topped with avocado salsa.

Vegetable and Tofu Coconut Curry

Ingredients:

- Firm tofu, cubed

- Mixed vegetables (bell peppers, snow peas, carrots)
- Coconut milk
- Red curry paste
- Onion, sliced
- Garlic, minced
- Ginger, grated
- Brown rice (optional)

Nutritional Information (Per Serving):

Calories	Protein	Fat	Carbohydrates
350	15g	20g	25g

Preparation Method:

1. Sauté tofu until lightly browned and set aside.
2. Sauté sliced onion, garlic, and ginger in a pan. Add red curry paste.
3. Add mixed vegetables and cook until tender.

4. Pour in coconut milk and add the tofu. Simmer for a few minutes and serve. Serve over brown rice if desired.

Grilled Vegetable Fajitas

Ingredients:

- Assorted bell peppers, sliced
- Red onion, sliced
- Zucchini, sliced
- Fajita seasoning
- Olive oil
- Whole grain or low-carb tortillas
- Avocado slices (optional)

Nutritional Information (Per Serving):

Calories	Protein	Fat	Carbohydrates
300	5g	10g	35g

Preparation Method:

1. Toss sliced vegetables with fajita seasoning and olive oil.

2. Grill until slightly charred and tender.

3. Serve in tortillas and top with avocado slices if desired.

Stuffed Bell Peppers with Turkey and Quinoa

Ingredients:

- Bell peppers
- Ground turkey
- Cooked quinoa
- Diced tomatoes
- Onion, diced
- Garlic, minced
- Italian seasoning
- Shredded cheese (optional)

Nutritional Information (Per Serving):

Calories	Protein	Fat	Carbohydrates

350	25g	12g	25g

Preparation Method:

1. Preheat the oven to 375°F (190°C).

2. Cut the tops off the bell peppers and remove seeds and membranes.

3. Cook ground turkey, onions, and garlic until browned. Add cooked quinoa, diced tomatoes, and Italian seasoning.

4. Stuff the peppers with the mixture, top with cheese if desired, and bake until the peppers are tender.

Baked Chicken with Asparagus and Parmesan

Ingredients:

- Chicken thighs or breasts
- Asparagus spears
- Olive oil
- Garlic powder

- Paprika

- Grated Parmesan cheese

- Lemon wedges (optional)

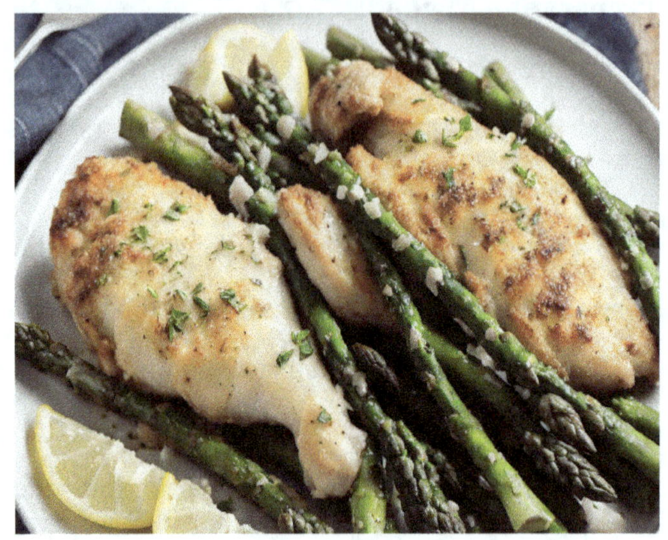

Nutritional Information (Per Serving):

Calories	Protein	Fat	Carbohydrates
300	30g	15g	5g

Preparation Method:

1. Preheat the oven to 400°F (200°C).

2. Rub chicken with olive oil, garlic powder, and paprika. Place in a baking dish.

3. Arrange asparagus around the chicken. Drizzle with olive oil and sprinkle with Parmesan cheese.

4. Bake until chicken is cooked and asparagus is tender. Serve with lemon wedges if desired.

Eggplant Lasagna

Ingredients:

- Eggplant, sliced lengthwise
- Ground turkey or beef
- Tomato sauce (low-sugar)
- Ricotta cheese
- Mozzarella cheese
- Basil leaves
- Italian seasoning, salt, and pepper

Nutritional Information (Per Serving):

Calories	Protein	Fat	Carbohydrates
250	20g	12g	15g

Preparation Method:

1. Preheat the oven to 375°F (190°C).

2. Grill or bake eggplant slices until slightly tender.

3. Cook ground meat with Italian seasoning, salt, and pepper. Add tomato sauce and simmer.

4. In a baking dish, layer eggplant, meat sauce, ricotta, mozzarella, and basil leaves. Repeat layers.

5. Bake until bubbly and golden.

Turkey Chili with Beans

Ingredients:

- Ground turkey
- Kidney beans, black beans
- Diced tomatoes

- Onion, diced

- Chili powder, cumin, paprika

- Garlic, minced

- Chicken or vegetable broth

Nutritional Information (Per Serving):

Calories	Protein	Fat	Carbohydrates
300	25g	10g	25g

Preparation Method:

1. Cook ground turkey with onion and garlic until browned.

2. Add diced tomatoes, beans, spices, and broth. Simmer for 20-30 minutes.

3. Adjust seasoning to taste and serve.

Lemon Herb Roasted Chicken Thighs

Ingredients:

- Chicken thighs, bone-in and skin-on

- Lemon juice

- Fresh herbs (rosemary, thyme)

- Garlic, minced

- Olive oil

- Salt and pepper

Nutritional Information (Per Serving):

Calories	Protein	Fat	Carbohydrates
350	25g	20g	2g

Preparation Method:

1. Preheat the oven to 400°F (200°C).

2. Combine lemon juice, herbs, garlic, olive oil, salt, and pepper.

3. Rub the chicken thighs with the mixture.

4. Roast in the oven until the internal temperature reaches 165°F (74°C).

Cauliflower Fried Rice with Tofu

Ingredients:

- Cauliflower rice

- Firm tofu, diced
- Mixed vegetables (peas, carrots, bell peppers)
- Soy sauce or tamari
- Sesame oil
- Minced ginger and garlic
- Scrambled eggs (optional)

Nutritional Information (Per Serving):

Calories	Protein	Fat	Carbohydrates
250	20g	15g	20g

Preparation Method:

1. Stir-fry diced tofu in sesame oil until browned. Set aside.
2. In the same pan, stir-fry mixed vegetables, ginger, and garlic.
3. Add cauliflower rice and soy sauce. Cook until heated through.

4. Add the cooked tofu back to the pan and scramble in eggs if desired.

Salmon Cakes with Avocado Aioli

Ingredients:

- Canned or cooked salmon

- Panko breadcrumbs

- Egg

- Diced red bell pepper

- Lemon zest

- Avocado, mashed

- Greek yogurt

- Garlic powder, salt, and pepper

Nutritional Information (Per Serving):

Calories	Protein	Fat	Carbohydrates
250	20g	15g	10g

Preparation Method:

1. Mix salmon, breadcrumbs, egg, bell pepper, lemon zest, and form into patties.
2. Pan-fry until golden brown.
3. For the aioli, mix mashed avocado, Greek yogurt, garlic powder, salt, and pepper.
4. Serve the salmon cakes with a dollop of avocado aioli.

Mushroom Stroganoff with Whole Wheat Pasta

Ingredients:
- Whole wheat pasta
- Mushrooms, sliced
- Onion, chopped
- Vegetable broth
- Greek yogurt or sour cream
- Paprika, thyme
- Olive oil
- Salt and pepper

Nutritional Information (Per Serving):

Calories	Protein	Fat	Carbohydrates
350	10g	10g	45g

Preparation Method:

1. Cook pasta according to package instructions.
2. Sauté mushrooms and onions in olive oil until tender.
3. Add vegetable broth, Greek yogurt or sour cream, paprika, and thyme.
4. Simmer until the sauce thickens. Serve over cooked whole wheat pasta.

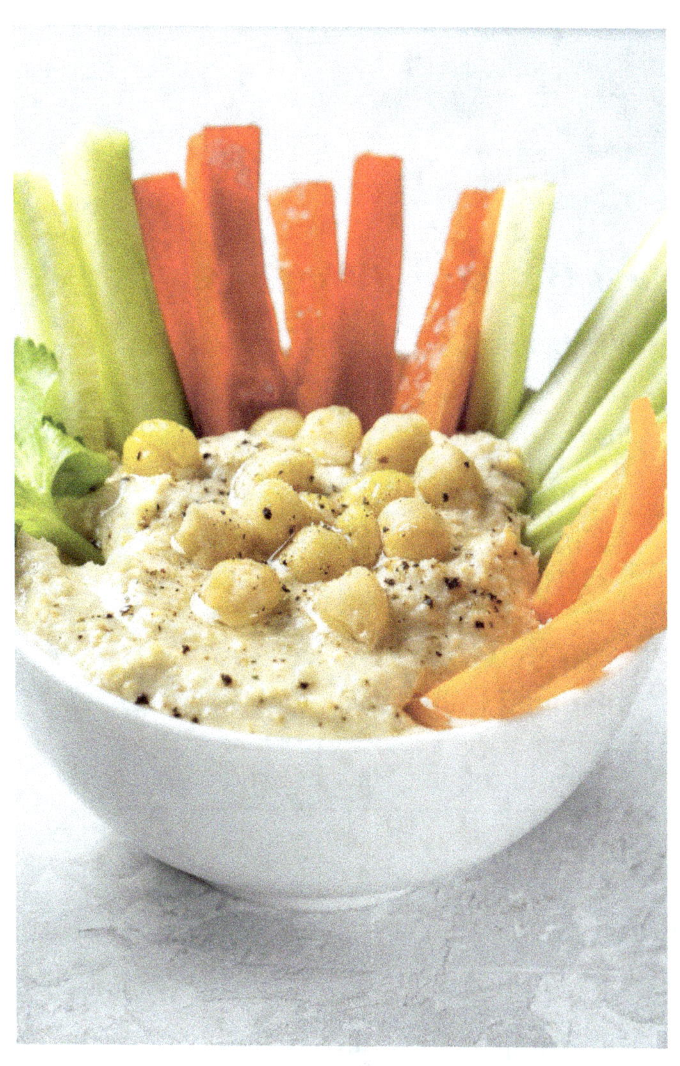

CHAPTER 6:

SNACKS AND SIDES

Veggie Sticks with Hummus

Ingredients:

- Carrot sticks
- Cucumber sticks
- Bell pepper strips
- Hummus (low-fat)

Nutritional Information (Per Serving):

Calories	Protein	Fat	Carbohydrates
150	3g	5g	15g

Preparation Method:

1. Simply slice the vegetables and serve with a portion of hummus for dipping.

Roasted Chickpeas

Ingredients:

- Canned chickpeas, drained and rinsed
- Olive oil
- Seasonings (such as paprika, cumin, garlic powder)
- Salt

Nutritional Information (Per Serving):

Calories	Protein	Fat	Carbohydrates
200	6g	4g	25g

Preparation Method:

1. Preheat the oven to 400°F (200°C).
2. Toss chickpeas with olive oil and seasonings.
3. Roast on a baking sheet for 25-30 minutes or until crunchy.

Avocado Deviled Eggs

Ingredients:

- Hard-boiled eggs, halved
- Ripe avocado
- Dijon mustard
- Lemon juice
- Chopped chives
- Salt and pepper

Nutritional Information (Per Serving):

Calories	Protein	Fat	Carbohydrates
100	6g	8g	3g

Preparation Method:

1. Scoop out egg yolks and mix with mashed avocado, mustard, lemon juice, chives, salt, and pepper.
2. Refill the egg whites with the avocado mixture.

Quinoa Tabbouleh Salad

Ingredients:

- Cooked quinoa
- Chopped fresh parsley
- Diced cucumber
- Diced tomatoes
- Lemon juice
- Olive oil
- Salt and pepper

Nutritional Information (Per Serving):

Calories	Protein	Fat	Carbohydrates
200	5g	8g	20g

Preparation Method:

1. Combine cooked quinoa, parsley, cucumber, and tomatoes.
2. Dress with lemon juice, olive oil, salt, and pepper.

Crispy Baked Zucchini Chips

Ingredients:

- Zucchini, thinly sliced
- Olive oil
- Parmesan cheese (optional)
- Garlic powder, salt, and pepper

Nutritional Information (Per Serving):

Calories	Protein	Fat	Carbohydrates
150	3g	8g	8g

Preparation Method:

1. Preheat the oven to 425°F (220°C).
2. Toss zucchini slices with olive oil, garlic powder, salt, and pepper.
3. Arrange on a baking sheet and bake until crispy. Sprinkle with Parmesan cheese if desired.

Cucumber and Tomato Salad

Ingredients:

- Sliced cucumbers
- Cherry tomatoes, halved
- Red onion, thinly sliced
- Fresh basil
- Balsamic vinegar
- Olive oil
- Salt and pepper

Nutritional Information (Per Serving):

Calories	Protein	Fat	Carbohydrates
100	2g	3g	8g

Preparation Method:

1. Toss sliced cucumbers, tomatoes, red onion, and torn basil in a bowl.
2. Dress with balsamic vinegar, olive oil, salt, and pepper.

Edamame with Sea Salt

Ingredients:

- Edamame (fresh or frozen)
- Sea salt

Nutritional Information (Per Serving):

Calories	Protein	Fat	Carbohydrates
150	10g	3g	10g

Preparation Method:

1. Boil or steam edamame according to package instructions.
2. Sprinkle it with sea salt and serve.

Stuffed Mini Bell Peppers

Ingredients:

- Mini bell peppers
- Light cream cheese or goat cheese
- Chopped chives or parsley
- Black pepper

Nutritional Information (Per Serving):

Calories	Protein	Fat	Carbohydrates
100	2g	3g	5g

Preparation Method:

1. Mix cream cheese or goat cheese with chopped chives or parsley.
2. Slice the tops off the mini bell peppers and remove seeds.
3. Stuff the peppers with the cheese mixture and sprinkle with black pepper.

Mango Salsa with Baked Pita Chips

Ingredients:

- Diced mango
- Diced red bell pepper
- Red onion, finely chopped
- Fresh cilantro
- Lime juice

- Whole grain pita bread
- Olive oil

Nutritional Information (Per Serving):

Calories	Protein	Fat	Carbohydrates
200	3g	4g	30g

Preparation Method:

1. Mix diced mango, red bell pepper, red onion, cilantro, and lime juice for the salsa.

2. Cut pita bread into triangles, brush with olive oil, and bake until crispy. Serve with the mango salsa.

Spicy Roasted Almonds

Ingredients:

- Raw almonds
- Olive oil
- Cayenne pepper

- Smoked paprika
- Sea salt

Nutritional Information (Per Serving):

Calories	Protein	Fat	Carbohydrates
150	6g	14g	6g

Preparation Method:

1. Preheat the oven to 325°F (160°C).
2. Toss almonds with olive oil, cayenne, paprika, and a pinch of salt.
3. Roast for 12-15 minutes until fragrant and crunchy.

Caprese Skewers

Ingredients:

- Cherry tomatoes
- Fresh mozzarella balls
- Basil leaves
- Balsamic glaze

- Skewers

Nutritional Information (Per Serving):

Calories	Protein	Fat	Carbohydrates
150	6g	7g	4g

Preparation Method:

1. Thread cherry tomatoes, mozzarella balls, and basil leaves onto skewers.
2. Drizzle with balsamic glaze before serving.

Roasted Red Pepper and Walnut Dip

Ingredients:

- Roasted red peppers (from a jar)
- Walnuts
- Garlic
- Lemon juice
- Olive oil
- Cumin, salt, and pepper

- Whole grain crackers or vegetable sticks

Nutritional Information (Per Serving):

Calories	Protein	Fat	Carbohydrates
150	2g	8g	6g

Preparation Method:

1. Blend red peppers, walnuts, garlic, lemon juice, olive oil, cumin, salt, and pepper until smooth.
2. Serve with whole grain crackers or veggie sticks.

Seaweed Snacks

Ingredients:

- Roasted seaweed sheets
- Sesame oil
- Soy sauce or tamari
- Sesame seeds

Nutritional Information (Per Serving):

Calories	Protein	Fat	Carbohydrates
100	2g	4g	1g

Preparation Method:

1. Lightly brush seaweed sheets with sesame oil and soy sauce.

2. Sprinkle with sesame seeds and cut into squares.

Cottage Cheese and Pineapple Cups

Ingredients:

- Cottage cheese
- Fresh pineapple, diced
- Mint leaves (optional)

Nutritional Information (Per Serving):

Calories	Protein	Fat	Carbohydrates
150	10g	2g	15g

Preparation Method:

1. Fill small cups or bowls with cottage cheese.

2. Top with diced pineapple and garnish with mint leaves, if desired.

Protein-Packed Tuna Salad

Ingredients:

- Canned tuna in water
- Greek yogurt
- Diced celery
- Diced red onion
- Dijon mustard
- Lemon juice
- Fresh dill
- Salt and pepper

Nutritional Information (Per Serving):

Calories	Protein	Fat	Carbohydrates

200	20g	3g	5g

Preparation Method:

1. Mix tuna, Greek yogurt, celery, red onion, Dijon mustard, lemon juice, dill, salt, and pepper in a bowl.

2. Serve on whole grain crackers or lettuce cups.

Spinach and Artichoke Stuffed Mushrooms

Ingredients:

- Mushrooms, stems removed
- Chopped spinach
- Chopped artichoke hearts
- Cream cheese or Greek yogurt
- Minced garlic
- Grated Parmesan cheese
- Salt and pepper

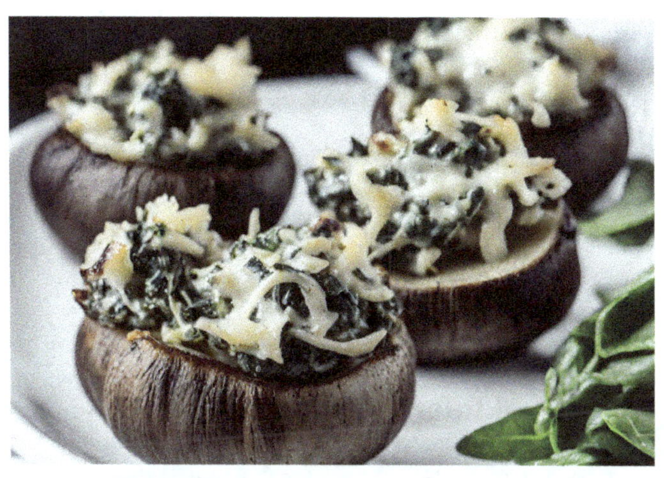

Nutritional Information (Per Serving):

Calories	Protein	Fat	Carbohydrates
150	5g	6g	8g

Preparation Method:

1. Preheat the oven to 375°F (190°C).

2. Mix spinach, artichokes, cream cheese or Greek yogurt, garlic, Parmesan, salt, and pepper.

3. Stuffed mushroom caps with the mixture and bake until golden.

Cinnamon Baked Apple Slices

Ingredients:

- Apple slices
- Cinnamon
- Raw honey (optional)
- Chopped nuts (almonds, walnuts)

Nutritional Information (Per Serving):

Calories	Protein	Fat	Carbohydrates
150	1g	3g	20g

Preparation Method:

1. Preheat the oven to 350°F (175°C).
2. Toss apple slices with cinnamon and honey if desired.
3. Bake until tender. Top with chopped nuts.

Quinoa and Black Bean Stuffed Mini Peppers

Ingredients:

- Mini bell peppers

- Cooked quinoa

- Black beans, rinsed and drained

- Salsa

- Shredded cheddar cheese

Nutritional Information (Per Serving):

Calories	Protein	Fat	Carbohydrates
200	6g	4g	25g

Preparation Method:

1. Cut the tops off the mini peppers and remove seeds.

2. Mix quinoa, black beans, salsa, and cheese.

3. Stuff the peppers and bake until the peppers are tender.

CHAPTER 7:

SWEET TREATS AND DESSERT DELIGHTS

Berry Yogurt Popsicles

Ingredients:

- Greek yogurt (unsweetened)
- Mixed berries (blueberries, strawberries, raspberries)
- Raw honey (optional)
- Vanilla extract

Nutritional Information (Per Serving):

Calories	Protein	Fat	Carbohydrates
70	3g	1g	8g

Preparation Method:

1. Blend Greek yogurt, berries, honey, and vanilla extract.

2. Pour the mixture into popsicle molds and freeze until solid.

Dark Chocolate Dipped Strawberries

Ingredients:

- Fresh strawberries
- Dark chocolate (70% or higher cocoa content)

Nutritional Information (Per Serving):

Calories	Protein	Fat	Carbohydrates
100	1g	3g	8g

Preparation Method:

1. Melt dark chocolate in a microwave or double boiler.

2. Dip each strawberry into the melted chocolate and place them on a parchment-lined tray to set.

Coconut and Almond Date Balls

Ingredients:

- Pitted dates
- Almonds
- Unsweetened shredded coconut
- Vanilla extract

Nutritional Information (Per Serving):

Calories	Protein	Fat	Carbohydrates
150	3g	5g	15g

Preparation Method:

1. Blend dates, almonds, coconut, and vanilla extract in a food processor.
2. Roll the mixture into balls and coat them with additional coconut if desired.

Frozen Banana Bites

Ingredients:

- Bananas, sliced
- Almond butter or peanut butter
- Unsweetened shredded coconut or chopped nuts

Nutritional Information (Per Serving):

Calories	Protein	Fat	Carbohydrates
100	1g	3g	10g

Preparation Method:

1. Spread almond or peanut butter between banana slices to create little sandwiches.
2. Roll the edges in shredded coconut or chopped nuts and freeze until firm.

Homemade Fruit Sorbet

Ingredients:

- Mixed frozen fruit (such as berries, mango, or pineapple)
- Fresh lemon or lime juice
- Raw honey or agave syrup (optional)

Nutritional Information (Per Serving):

Calories	Protein	Fat	Carbohydrates
80	1g	0g	15g

Preparation Method:

1. Blend the frozen fruit with citrus juice and sweetener if desired until smooth.
2. Freeze for a few hours until firm or serve immediately.

Yogurt and Fresh Fruit Parfait

Ingredients:

- Greek yogurt (unsweetened)
- Fresh mixed fruits (berries, sliced peaches, or kiwi)

- Granola (sugar-free or low-sugar)
- Raw honey or maple syrup (optional)

Nutritional Information (Per Serving):

Calories	Protein	Fat	Carbohydrates
150	5g	2g	20g

Preparation Method:

1. Layer Greek yogurt, mixed fruits, and granola in a glass or bowl.
2. Drizzle with honey or maple syrup for added sweetness if desired.

Baked Apple Chips

Ingredients:

- Apples, thinly sliced
- Cinnamon
- Raw honey (optional)

Nutritional Information (Per Serving):

Calories	Protein	Fat	Carbohydrates
100	0g	0g	15g

Preparation Method:

1. Preheat the oven to 200°F (95°C).

2. Arrange apple slices on a baking sheet, sprinkle with cinnamon and honey, and bake until dried and slightly crisp.

Frozen Yogurt Bark

Ingredients:

- Greek yogurt (unsweetened)
- Fresh berries (blueberries, raspberries)
- Sliced almonds or shredded coconut
- Raw honey or maple syrup (optional)

Nutritional Information (Per Serving):

Calories	Protein	Fat	Carbohydrates
70	3g	2g	10g

Preparation Method:

1. Line a baking sheet with parchment paper and spread yogurt evenly.

2. Top with berries, nuts, and a drizzle of honey or maple syrup.

3. Freeze until firm, then break into pieces.

Chocolate Avocado Mousse

Ingredients:

- Ripe avocados

- Unsweetened cocoa powder

- Raw honey or maple syrup

- Vanilla extract

Nutritional Information (Per Serving):

Calories	Protein	Fat	Carbohydrates
150	2g	8g	10g

Preparation Method:

1. Blend avocados, cocoa powder, sweetener, and vanilla until smooth and creamy.
2. Chill before serving.

Protein-Rich Banana Oat Cookies

Ingredients:

- Ripe bananas, mashed
- Rolled oats
- Whey protein powder (unsweetened)
- Cinnamon
- Raisins or chopped nuts (optional)

Nutritional Information (Per Serving):

Calories	Protein	Fat	Carbohydrates
100	4g	1g	10g

Preparation Method:

1. Preheat the oven to 350°F (175°C).

2. Mix mashed bananas, oats, protein powder, cinnamon, and any additional ingredients.

3. Spoon onto a baking sheet and bake until golden.

Vanilla Almond Butter Fudge

Ingredients:

- Almond butter (unsweetened)
- Coconut oil
- Vanilla extract
- Raw honey or maple syrup (optional)

Nutritional Information (Per Serving):

Calories	Protein	Fat	Carbohydrates
100	3g	10g	5g

Preparation Method:

1. Melt almond butter and coconut oil together. Stir in vanilla and sweetener if desired.

2. Pour the mixture into a pan lined with parchment paper and freeze until solid.

CHAPTER 8:

CONCLUSION

Essential Cooking Techniques

1. **Grilling and Broiling:** Use these methods for lean proteins like fish, chicken, and turkey. Season with herbs and spices rather than heavy sauces.

2. **Steaming:** Ideal for vegetables to retain their nutrients. Steaming helps preserve their natural flavors without adding extra fats.

3. **Sauteing with Healthy Oils:** Use heart-healthy oils like olive oil, avocado oil, or coconut oil for sautéing vegetables or lean proteins. Add garlic and herbs for flavor.

4. **Roasting and Baking:** Roast or bake vegetables, such as cauliflower, broccoli,

and sweet potatoes, to bring out their natural sweetness without the need for added fats.

5. **Preparing Homemade Dressings and Sauces:** Make your own dressings and sauces using ingredients like olive oil, lemon juice, fresh herbs, and natural sweeteners like honey or maple syrup. This helps avoid the added sugars and preservatives found in many store-bought versions.

6. **Low-Sodium Broths and Stocks:** Utilize low-sodium or homemade broths and stocks for soups and stews. They add flavor without excessive sodium, maintaining the diet's principles.

7. **Herb and Spice Seasoning:** Enhance flavor using various herbs and spices instead of salt or high-sodium seasonings. Experiment with

combinations like oregano, thyme, basil, and turmeric for added health benefits.

8. **Whole Grains Preparation:** Cook whole grains like quinoa, brown rice, and farro using the absorption or pilaf method to maintain their texture and nutritional content.

9. **Healthy Dessert Alternatives:** Explore baking with natural sweeteners like dates, honey, or maple syrup to create healthier dessert options. Utilize almond flour or oats for crusts and bases.

10. **Creative Salad Making:** Construct salads with a variety of vegetables, leafy greens, nuts, seeds, and lean proteins. Experiment with homemade vinaigrettes for added flavor.

11. **Mindful Portion Control:** Pay attention to portion sizes to maintain a balanced intake. Practice mindful eating to prevent overeating.

12. **Experimentation and Creativity:** Be open to experimenting with new ingredients, flavors, and recipes that align with the Galveston Diet principles. This can keep meals interesting and varied.

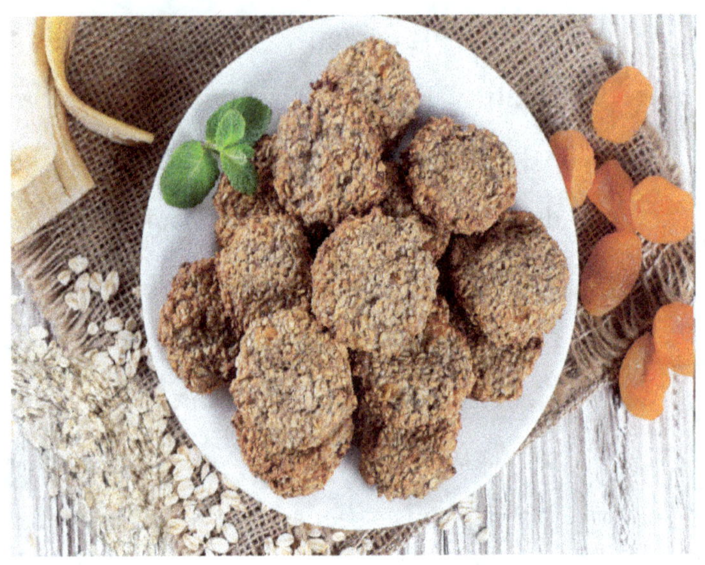

Attention Galveston Diet Cookbook readers! Your feedback matters! If you've explored the nutritious recipes and insightful guidance within this cookbook, we'd love to hear from you.

Your reviews help others discover the benefits and flavors awaiting them. Share your experience, thoughts, and how the Galveston Diet Cookbook has influenced your health journey. Your review could be the inspiration someone needs to embark on a path toward a healthier lifestyle. Your words make a difference! Take a moment to review the Galveston Diet Cookbook and let your voice shape the culinary journeys of others. Thank you for being a part of this enriching experience!

www.ingramcontent.com/pod-product-compliance
Lightning Source LLC
Chambersburg PA
CBHW070945260726
48661CB00003B/1126